TRICYCLIC ANTIDEPRESSANTS

"Exploring The Legacy And Contemporary Utility Of A Classic Pharmacological Approach"

Mary J. Anderson

Table of Contents

"Unlocking the Power of Tricyclic Antidepressants: Mechanisms, Applications, and Considerations" 1

  "Exploring the Legacy and Contemporary Utility of a Classic Pharmacological Approach" 1

    Abstract..................................2

    Introduction 4

Chapter One..................................10

  Introduction to Tricyclic Antidepressants 10

  Authentic Setting: 11

  Synthetic Construction and Pharmacology: 12

  Clinical Applications: 13

  Difficulties and Contemplations: 14

Chapter Two..................................17

  Pharmacokinetics of Tricyclic Antidepressants 17

  Absorption: 18

  Distribution: 19

  Metabolism: 20

  Excretion: 22

Factors Impacting Pharmacokinetics: ...23

Clinical Ramifications: 25

Chapter Three..27

Efficacy and Clinical Effectiveness.........27

Viability in Sorrow: 28

Near Adequacy: 29

Signs Past Misery:...................................31

Factors Affecting Treatment Reaction:..32

Treatment Rules and Suggestions: 33

Chapter Four 36

Side Effects and Adverse Reactions of Tricyclic Antidepressants (TCAs) 36

Normal Incidental effects:......................37

Anticholinergic Impacts:............................37

Sedation:...37

Orthostatic Hypotension: 38

Weight Gain: 38

Cardiovascular Impacts: 39

QT Prolongation:..39

Heart Conduction Irregularities: 39

Neurological Impacts:............................40

Mental Impedance:.....................................40

Extrapyramidal Side effects: 40
    Mental Impacts: 41
Actuation and Tumult: 41
Madness or Hypomania: 41
    Gastrointestinal Impacts: 41
Sexual Brokenness: 42
Antagonistic Responses: 42
Drug Connections: 44
Checking and The executives: 45
Chapter Five 48
    Clinical Considerations and Special Populations................48
    Dosing Contemplations 49
Beginning Dosing: 49
Upkeep Dosing: 49
Individualized Treatment 50
Cardiovascular Impacts: 50
    Drug Connections: 52
a. Youngsters and Teenagers: 53
b. Old People: 54
c. Pregnant Ladies: 55
    Comorbid Ailments: 56

Chapter Six 59
    Monitoring and Safety 59
    Standard Appraisals: 60

Extensive Assessment: 60

Actual Assessment: 60

Lab Examinations: 61

Continuous Observing: 61

Antagonistic Impacts: 62

Security Observing: 63

Security Insurances: 64

Electrocardiographic Checking: 65

    The executives of Unfriendly Occasions: 66

Suggestive Treatment: 66

Portion Change: 66

Drug Connections: 67

Patient Instruction and Directing: 68

Chapter Seven 71
    Switching and Discontinuation 71
    Signs for Exchanging or Stopping: 72

Lacking Reaction: 72

Aftereffects: 72

Drug Connections: 73
Patient Inclination: 73
   Methodologies for Exchanging: 74
Cross-Tapering:..74
Monitoring:..75
The executives of Withdrawal Side effects:
....76
Contemplations for Elective Medicines:....78
Patient Instruction and Directing: 80
Chapter Eight..83
   Drug Interactions and Contraindications
....83
   Instruments of Medication Connections:
....84
Pharmacokinetic Cooperations: 84
Pharmacodynamic Collaborations: 85
   Normal Medication Communications:..86
a. Cytochrome P450 Inhibitors: 86
b. Cytochrome P450 Inducers: 87
c. Anticholinergic Specialists: 87
d. Cardiovascular Prescriptions: 88
e. Monoamine Oxidase Inhibitors (MAOIs):
....89

Contraindications: 90

a. Extreme touchiness: 90

b. Intense Recuperation 90

c. Accompanying Use with MAOIs: 90

d. Point Conclusion Glaucoma: 91

The board Systems: 91

Portion Change: 92

Monitoring: 92

Chapter Nine 96

Patient Education and Counseling in Tricyclic Antidepressant (TCA) Therapy 96

Significance of Patient Instruction: 97

a. Treatment Getting it: 97

c. Adherence Advancement: 98

d. Side effect Acknowledgment: 99

e. Self-Administration Abilities: 99

Key Parts of Patient Schooling: 100

a. Individualized Approach: 100

b. Clear Correspondence: 100

c. Intelligent Learning: 101

d. Support of Inquiries: 101

e. Support: 102

Directing Techniques: 102
b. Psychosocial Evaluation: 103
c. Psychoeducation: 103
d. Mental Conduct Procedures: 104
e. Backslide Anticipation: 104
Job of Medical services Suppliers: 105
a. Patient-Focused Care: 105
b. Social Responsiveness: 105
c. Coherence of Care: 106
Chapter Ten 109
Future Directions and Research 109
Pharmacological Advancements: 110
a. Novel TCA Subsidiaries: 110
b. Designated Medication 111
Customized Medication Approaches: ...112
a. Pharmacogenomics: 112
b. Biomarkers: 112
Novel Treatment Techniques: 113
a. Mix Treatments: 113
b. Increase Systems: 114
Advanced Wellbeing Intercessions: 115
a. Portable Wellbeing 115

b. Telepsychiatry: 115
    Neurobiological Components: 116
a. Neuroinflammation: 116
b. Brain adaptability: 117
    Relative Adequacy Exploration: 118
a. Similar Adequacy and Bearableness: ...118
b. Long haul Results: 118

Abstract

Tricyclic antidepressants (TCAs) represent a class of medications that have been pivotal in the treatment of depression and various psychiatric disorders for decades.

Despite the advent of newer antidepressant classes, TCAs continue to hold relevance due to their efficacy in managing symptoms and diverse mechanisms of action. By inhibiting the reuptake of neurotransmitters such as serotonin and norepinephrine, TCAs modulate mood and alleviate depressive symptoms.

However, their use is often tempered by a range of side effects and potential complications, necessitating careful patient selection and monitoring.

Understanding the nuanced pharmacology and clinical considerations surrounding TCAs remains paramount in contemporary psychiatric practice.

Introduction

Tricyclic antidepressants (TCAs) address a foundation throughout the entire existence of psychopharmacology, denoting a critical progression in the treatment of melancholy and other mental problems. Presented during the 1950s, TCAs reformed the administration of temperament problems by offering a pharmacological methodology particular from prior medicines like electroconvulsive treatment and therapy. The disclosure of imipramine, the prototypical TCA, proclaimed another period in mental therapeutics and made ready for ensuing medication advancement endeavors.

TCAs get their name from their tricyclic synthetic design, described by three rings combined. This special sub-atomic arrangement gives their pharmacological properties, including hindrance of the reuptake of synapses like serotonin and norepinephrine. By obstructing the presynaptic reuptake siphons, TCAs increment the synaptic centralizations of these synapses, in this manner upgrading neurotransmission and adjusting temperament.

The adequacy of TCAs in treating sadness comes from their capacity to reestablish the equilibrium of synapses inside the mind, especially in regions embroiled in temperament guideline. Serotonin and norepinephrine assume vital parts in tweaking profound states, and modifications in their levels have been ensnared in the pathophysiology of despondency. By upgrading serotonergic and noradrenergic neurotransmission, TCAs lighten burdensome side effects and work on generally working.

In spite of their viability, TCAs are related with a scope of aftereffects and security concerns, originating from their wide pharmacological consequences for different synapse frameworks. Normal aftereffects incorporate anticholinergic impacts (e.g., dry mouth, stoppage, obscured vision), sedation, weight gain, orthostatic hypotension, and heart conduction anomalies. Moreover, TCAs convey a gamble of excess related harmfulness, with possibly perilous outcomes like cardiotoxicity and seizures.

As of late, the coming of more current classes of

antidepressants, like particular serotonin reuptake inhibitors (SSRIs) and serotonin-norepinephrine reuptake inhibitors (SNRIs), has prompted a decrease in the utilization of TCAs as first-line medicines for discouragement. Be that as it may, TCAs keep on holding significance in specific clinical situations, especially in people who have not answered other energizer classes or who require expansion systems for treatment-safe despondency.

In this complete audit, we will investigate the pharmacology, viability, secondary effect profile, clinical contemplations, and contemporary utilizations of TCAs in the administration of despondency and other mental issues. By diving into the rich history and current utility of TCAs, we intend to give clinicians and scientists a nuanced comprehension of this persevering through class of antidepressants.

Chapter One

Introduction to Tricyclic Antidepressants

Tricyclic antidepressants (TCAs) stand as a trademark throughout the entire existence of psychopharmacology, addressing a critical headway in the treatment of despondency and related mental issues. This class of meds, described by their tricyclic synthetic construction, plays had a significant impact in forming the scene of present day mental pharmacotherapy. Understanding the presentation and advancement of TCAs is fundamental to see the value in their effect on clinical practice and patient consideration.

Authentic Setting:

The improvement of TCAs can be followed back to the mid-twentieth 100 years, when the treatment of psychological sickness depended overwhelmingly on psychotherapeutic methodologies and unrefined pharmacological mediations. The disclosure of imipramine during the 1950s denoted a defining moment in the field, proclaiming the rise of another class of energizer prescriptions. Imipramine, the prototypical TCA, was at first blended as a likely antipsychotic however was fortunately found to have state of mind hoisting properties.

Synthetic Construction and Pharmacology:

Tricyclic antidepressants get their name from the tricyclic ring structure shared by all individuals from this class. This one of a kind compound plan, containing three intertwined rings, bestows pharmacological properties that recognize TCAs from other stimulant classes. The essential instrument of activity of TCAs includes the hindrance of the reuptake of synapses like serotonin and norepinephrine, consequently expanding their synaptic focuses. This upgrade of neurotransmission is accepted to underlie the stimulant impacts of TCAs.

Clinical Applications:

TCAs have shown viability in the treatment of different mental problems, with significant burdensome issue (MDD) being the most deeply grounded sign. Furthermore, TCAs have been utilized to oversee conditions, for example, summed up tension turmoil (Stray), alarm jumble, fanatical urgent issue (OCD), neuropathic torment disorders, and nighttime enuresis in kids. Regardless of the appearance of more current energizer classes, TCAs keep on being endorsed in specific clinical situations, especially when different medicines have demonstrated inadequate or are contraindicated.

Difficulties and Contemplations:

While TCAs have contributed essentially to the treatment of discouragement and related conditions, their clinical utility is tempered by a scope of difficulties and contemplations. TCAs are related with a significant weight of secondary effects, including anticholinergic impacts, sedation, orthostatic hypotension, and cardiotoxicity. Additionally, the thin restorative record of TCAs requires cautious dosing and observing to stay away from harmfulness. Also, TCAs might connect with various drugs and require alert in patients with specific ailments.

In outline, the presentation of tricyclic antidepressants addressed a turning point in the field of psychiatry, offering a pharmacological methodology that changed the treatment of despondency and related messes. Notwithstanding their constraints,

TCAs keep on possessing an unmistakable spot in the armamentarium of mental therapeutics, highlighting their persevering through importance in present day clinical practice. Figuring out the authentic setting, substance properties, pharmacological instruments, clinical applications, and difficulties related with TCAs is fundamental for clinicians and scientists the same as they explore the intricacies of mental treatment.

Chapter Two

Pharmacokinetics of Tricyclic Antidepressants

Tricyclic antidepressants (TCAs) are a class of drugs that have been utilized for a really long time in the treatment of discouragement and other mental issues. Understanding the pharmacokinetics of TCAs is fundamental for streamlining their helpful viability, limiting antagonistic impacts, and guaranteeing protected and successful use in clinical practice. This far reaching outline will investigate the key pharmacokinetic boundaries of

TCAs, including retention, dissemination, digestion, and discharge, as well as variables impacting their pharmacokinetic profile and clinical ramifications.

Absorption:
The retention of TCAs basically happens in the gastrointestinal plot after oral organization. In any case, the rate and degree of retention can shift fundamentally among individual TCAs because of contrasts in their compound properties, like lipophilicity and dissolvability. Factors like gastric pH, food admission, and plan qualities (e.g., quick delivery versus broadened

discharge) can impact TCA assimilation. Some TCAs, for example, amitriptyline and imipramine, show unpredictable ingestion examples and variable bioavailability, while others, similar to nortriptyline and desipramine, are all the more promptly retained.

Distribution:

Upon ingestion, TCAs are broadly disseminated all through the body, including into different tissues and organs. TCAs are exceptionally lipophilic mixtures, which works with their entrance across organic films and dispersion into tissues past the circulation system. Protein restricting, principally to egg whites, fundamentally impacts the conveyance of TCAs in the plasma. The level of protein restricting differs among individual TCAs, with some showing high protein restricting (>90%) and others showing lower protein restricting fondness. This protein-bound part fills in as a supply for TCAs, impacting their pharmacokinetic profile and span of activity.

Metabolism:

Digestion assumes a vital part in the biotransformation of TCAs, basically happening in the liver through hepatic chemical frameworks, especially the cytochrome P450 (CYP) protein family. TCAs go through oxidative digestion, fundamentally by means of the CYP2D6 and CYP2C19 isoenzymes, bringing about the arrangement of dynamic and inert metabolites. The metabolic pathways of individual TCAs can fluctuate, prompting contrasts in their pharmacokinetic profiles and potential for drug communications. Hereditary polymorphisms in CYP catalysts can likewise add to interindividual changeability in TCA digestion, impacting drug viability and harmfulness.

Excretion:

The end of TCAs and their metabolites happens fundamentally through renal discharge, with a more modest portion discharged in defecation. Renal discharge includes both glomerular filtration and dynamic cylindrical emission, with the kidneys assuming an overwhelming part in TCA freedom from the body. The pharmacokinetics of TCAs are impacted by renal capability, with disabled renal capability prompting diminished drug freedom and delayed disposal half-life. Portion changes might be important in patients with renal weakness to keep away from drug gathering and limit the gamble of unfriendly impacts.

Factors Impacting Pharmacokinetics:

A few elements can impact the pharmacokinetics of TCAs, including age, hepatic capability, renal capability, hereditary polymorphisms, drug collaborations, and patient-explicit qualities. Old people might display adjusted pharmacokinetics because old enough related changes in drug digestion and leeway. Hepatic hindrance can influence TCA digestion, prompting expanded plasma fixations and likely poisonousness. Essentially, renal debilitation can impede drug end, requiring portion changes in accordance with forestall drug aggregation. Hereditary polymorphisms in CYP chemicals can bring about changeability in drug digestion among people, affecting TCA viability and security. Drug communications with inhibitors or inducers of CYP catalysts can likewise adjust TCA digestion and pharmacokinetics, prompting expected unfavorable impacts or restorative disappointment.

Clinical Ramifications:

A comprehension of the pharmacokinetics of TCAs has significant clinical ramifications for their utilization in mental practice. Clinicians should consider factors like medication retention, conveyance, digestion, and discharge while choosing TCA details, deciding dosing regimens, and checking patients during treatment. Individual patient qualities, including age, hepatic capability, renal capability, and hereditary changeability, ought to likewise be considered to upgrade TCA treatment and limit the gamble of unfriendly impacts or treatment disappointment.

In rundown, the pharmacokinetics of tricyclic antidepressants assume a significant part in deciding their remedial viability, security, and clinical utility in the treatment of misery and related mental issues. By figuring out the ingestion, circulation, digestion, and discharge of TCAs, clinicians can settle on informed choices in regards to sedate determination, dosing, and checking, eventually improving patient consideration and treatment results.

Chapter Three

Efficacy and Clinical Effectiveness

Tricyclic antidepressants (TCAs) have been a backbone in the treatment of discouragement and other mental problems for a really long time. Notwithstanding the rise of more up to date energizer classes, TCAs keep on being endorsed because of their laid out viability in overseeing burdensome side effects. Understanding the adequacy and clinical viability of TCAs is fundamental for directing treatment choices and upgrading patient results. This far reaching outline will investigate the proof supporting the utilization of TCAs, remembering their viability for wretchedness and different signs, relative adequacy, and elements impacting treatment reaction.

Viability in Sorrow:

Various clinical preliminaries and meta-examinations have exhibited the adequacy of TCAs in the treatment of significant burdensome problem (MDD). TCAs have shown equivalent viability to fresher upper classes, like specific serotonin reuptake inhibitors (SSRIs), in lightening burdensome side effects and accomplishing abatement. Studies have demonstrated the way that TCAs can create huge enhancements in temperament, rest, craving, and generally speaking working in patients with misery. In any case, the beginning of activity of TCAs might be more slow contrasted with fresher antidepressants, with a little while regularly expected to accomplish restorative impacts.

Near Adequacy:

Near viability review have analyzed the general adequacy of TCAs contrasted with other upper classes, like SSRIs, serotonin-norepinephrine reuptake inhibitors (SNRIs), and monoamine oxidase inhibitors (MAOIs). While TCAs have shown practically identical viability to SSRIs and SNRIs in treating sorrow, they might be related with a higher weight of secondary effects and wellbeing concerns. MAOIs, one more class of more seasoned antidepressants, have shown comparative viability to TCAs yet are held for use in hard-headed cases because of their true capacity for serious medication collaborations and dietary limitations.

Signs Past Misery:

Notwithstanding misery, TCAs have been utilized in the therapy of different mental and ailments. TCAs have shown adequacy in overseeing uneasiness issues, for example, alarm jumble, summed up nervousness jumble (Stray), and fanatical enthusiastic problem (OCD). They are additionally involved off-name for conditions, for example, neuropathic torment disorders, headaches, and nighttime enuresis in kids. The expansive pharmacological impacts of TCAs, including their adjustment of synapse frameworks past serotonin and norepinephrine, add to their viability across various signs.

Factors Affecting Treatment Reaction:

A few elements can impact individual reactions to TCA therapy, including hereditary variables, pharmacokinetic fluctuation, comorbid ailments, and psychosocial factors. Hereditary polymorphisms in drug-using compounds, like CYP2D6 and CYP2C19, can influence TCA digestion and plasma fixations, impacting treatment reaction and decency. Patients with comorbid ailments, like cardiovascular infection or hepatic debilitation, may require portion changes or closer checking because of possible communications or unfavorable impacts.

Treatment Rules and Suggestions:

Clinical practice rules give proposals to the utilization of TCAs in the administration of sorrow and related conditions. These rules normally stress the significance of individualized treatment draws near, taking into account factors like side effect seriousness, treatment history, patient inclinations, and wellbeing concerns. While TCAs stay a suitable treatment choice for certain patients, especially the people who have not answered other stimulant classes, their utilization might be restricted by decency issues and wellbeing contemplations.

All in all, tricyclic antidepressants (TCAs) keep on assuming a critical part in the treatment of sadness and other mental issues, showing viability equivalent to more current upper classes. Be that as it may, their utilization is in many cases tempered by a higher weight of secondary effects and security concerns. Understanding the proof supporting the viability and clinical adequacy of TCAs, as well as variables affecting treatment reaction, is fundamental for informed direction and ideal patient consideration in mental practice.

Chapter Four

Side Effects and Adverse Reactions of Tricyclic Antidepressants (TCAs)

Tricyclic antidepressants (TCAs) have been broadly utilized in the treatment of sadness and other mental issues for quite a long time. While successful in overseeing burdensome side effects, TCAs are related with a scope of secondary effects and unfavorable responses that can restrict their decency and adherence. Understanding the expected aftereffects and unfavorable responses of TCAs is fundamental for clinicians to go with informed treatment choices and screen patients for security and viability.

Normal Incidental effects:

Anticholinergic Impacts: TCAs apply anticholinergic impacts by hindering muscarinic acetylcholine receptors, prompting side effects like dry mouth, obscured vision, clogging, urinary maintenance, and mental disability.

Sedation: TCAs can cause sedation and tiredness, which might obstruct day to day exercises and add to exhaustion and daytime languor.

Orthostatic Hypotension: TCAs can prompt a drop in circulatory strain after standing (orthostatic hypotension), prompting discombobulation, dazedness, and blacking out.

Weight Gain: Some TCAs, like amitriptyline and imipramine, are related with weight gain, which can add to metabolic unsettling influences and effect patients' confidence and adherence to treatment.

Cardiovascular Impacts:

QT Prolongation: TCAs can draw out the QT stretch on electrocardiogram (ECG), which might build the gamble of ventricular arrhythmias, including torsades de pointes, especially at higher dosages.

Heart Conduction Irregularities: TCAs can disturb cardiovascular conduction, prompting sinus tachycardia, atrioventricular block, and group branch block, which might encourage heart arrhythmias.

Neurological Impacts:

Mental Impedance: TCAs can debilitate mental capability, including memory, consideration, and chief capability, which might affect patients' capacity to perform everyday undertakings and keep up with social and word related working.

Extrapyramidal Side effects: TCAs might prompt extrapyramidal side effects, like quakes, dystonia, and dyskinesias, looking like those seen with antipsychotic prescriptions.

Mental Impacts:
Actuation and Tumult: TCAs may oddly actuate enactment and fomentation in certain patients, appearing as fretfulness, touchiness, and sleep deprivation.

Madness or Hypomania: TCAs can encourage hyper or hypomanic episodes in people with bipolar confusion or an inclination to bipolar range problems.

Gastrointestinal Impacts:
Gastrointestinal Unsettling influences: TCAs might cause gastrointestinal secondary effects, including sickness, spewing,

looseness of the bowels, and stomach distress, which can influence patients' personal satisfaction and adherence to therapy.

Sexual Brokenness:
TCAs can initiate sexual brokenness, including diminished moxie, erectile brokenness, and deferred discharge, which may unfavorably influence patients' personal connections and generally prosperity.

Antagonistic Responses:
Serotonin Disorder: In uncommon cases, TCAs can

encourage serotonin disorder, a possibly dangerous condition described by hyperthermia, fomentation, quake, and autonomic unsteadiness, coming about because of exorbitant serotoninergic action.

Extreme touchiness Responses: TCAs can seldom cause hypersensitive responses, including skin rashes, pruritus, angioedema, and hypersensitivity, requiring quick clinical consideration and end of the culpable specialist.

Drug Connections:

TCAs can collaborate with various meds, including other psychotropic specialists, cardiovascular meds, and medications influencing cytochrome P450 chemicals, prompting potential pharmacokinetic and pharmacodynamic cooperations.

Corresponding utilization of TCAs with monoamine oxidase inhibitors (MAOIs) can bring about serotonin condition or hypertensive emergency, requiring a waste of time period between end of MAOIs and commencement of TCAs.

Checking and The executives:
Clinicians ought to screen patients getting TCAs for the development of secondary effects and unfavorable responses, especially during the underlying long stretches of treatment and following portion changes.

The executives systems for TCAs' aftereffects incorporate portion decrease, changing to elective meds, indicative therapy, and tending to modifiable gamble factors, like way of life adjustments and comorbid ailments.

Patient instruction and guiding are fundamental to illuminate patients about the likely aftereffects and antagonistic responses of TCAs, elevate adherence to treatment, and engage patients to report side effects expeditiously for ideal mediation.

In outline, tricyclic antidepressants (TCAs) are related with a range of secondary effects and unfavorable responses that can affect patients' decency, adherence, and security. Clinicians ought to painstakingly consider the gamble benefit profile of TCAs and screen patients intently for the rise of incidental effects and unfriendly responses. Individualized treatment draws near, patient training, and proactive administration techniques are fundamental to streamline the remedial advantages of TCAs while limiting their likely dangers.

Chapter Five

Clinical Considerations and Special Populations

Tricyclic antidepressants (TCAs) have been used for quite a long time in the treatment of misery and other mental issues. While powerful, their utilization requires cautious thought of different clinical elements and unique populaces to improve remedial results and limit chances. This far reaching outline will investigate the clinical contemplations related with TCA treatment, including dosing contemplations, wellbeing concerns, and extraordinary populaces like kids, youths, older people, and pregnant ladies.

Dosing Contemplations

Beginning Dosing: Commencement of TCA treatment ordinarily includes beginning with low dosages and continuously titrating vertically to accomplish remedial adequacy while limiting incidental effects. The underlying portion might be lower in old patients and those with clinical comorbidities.

Upkeep Dosing: When helpful reaction is accomplished, TCAs are normally managed at support dosages to support abatement and forestall backslide. Upkeep dosing may shift in light of individual patient attributes, side effect seriousness, and treatment reaction.

Individualized Treatment: TCAs ought to be individualized in light of patient-explicit elements, including age, weight, renal capability, hepatic capability, attending drugs, and comorbid ailments. Close observing and portion changes might be important to advance treatment results.

Cardiovascular Impacts: TCAs are related with

cardiovascular secondary effects, including orthostatic hypotension, QT prolongation, and conduction irregularities. Alert is justified in patients with previous cardiovascular circumstances, like arrhythmias, ischemic coronary illness, or cardiovascular breakdown.

Self destruction Hazard: TCAs convey a black box cautioning with respect to the expanded gamble of self-destructive ideation and conduct, especially in kids, teenagers, and youthful grown-ups. Close observing for suicidality is fundamental during the underlying long stretches of treatment and following portion changes.

Drug Connections: TCAs can cooperate with various prescriptions, including other psychotropic specialists, cardiovascular meds, and medications influencing cytochrome P450 proteins, prompting potential pharmacokinetic and pharmacodynamic associations. Clinicians ought to assess potential medication connections and change TCA dosing or consider elective treatments on a case by case basis.

a. Youngsters and Teenagers:

TCAs are for the most part not suggested as first-line treatment for pediatric melancholy because of security concerns and the accessibility of more secure other options.

Use in kids and teenagers ought to be saved for cases stubborn to different medicines, and close observing for unfavorable impacts, including suicidality, is fundamental.

b. Old People:

Older patients might be more vulnerable to unfriendly impacts of TCAs, including anticholinergic impacts, sedation, and orthostatic hypotension, because old enough related changes in drug digestion and leeway.

Lower starting dosages and more slow titration might be justified in old patients to limit aftereffects and decrease the gamble of falls and mental hindrance.

c. Pregnant Ladies:

TCAs are for the most part viewed as somewhat ok for use during pregnancy, in spite of the fact that information on their security in pregnancy are restricted.

TCAs ought to be utilized with alert during pregnancy, especially during the principal trimester when organogenesis happens, and the most reduced successful portion ought to be utilized to limit fetal openness.

Close observing for neonatal withdrawal side effects and

possible unfriendly impacts on fetal advancement is suggested.

Comorbid Ailments:

TCAs ought to be utilized warily in patients with comorbid ailments, like cardiovascular sickness, hepatic hindrance, renal debilitation, and seizure problems, as these circumstances might expand the gamble of antagonistic impacts or confuse therapy.

Close checking and portion changes might be fundamental in patients with comorbid ailments to guarantee wellbeing and adequacy.

In rundown, the utilization of tricyclic antidepressants (TCAs) requires cautious thought of clinical variables and exceptional populaces to upgrade treatment results and limit chances. Clinicians ought to individualize TCA treatment in light of patient-explicit attributes, intently screen for unfavorable impacts, and exercise alert in unique populaces like youngsters, teenagers, older people, and pregnant ladies. Via cautiously gauging the advantages and dangers of TCA treatment and carrying out fitting checking and the executives methodologies, clinicians can upgrade the security and adequacy of TCA treatment in different patient populaces.

Chapter Six

Monitoring and Safety

Tricyclic antidepressants (TCAs) have been broadly utilized in the treatment of sadness and other mental issues for quite a long time. While successful, their utilization requires tenacious checking and thoughtfulness regarding wellbeing contemplations to limit the gamble of unfriendly impacts and upgrade treatment results. This far reaching outline will investigate the fundamental parts of checking and security in TCA treatment, including benchmark evaluations, continuous observing, wellbeing precautionary measures, and the board of likely unfriendly occasions.

Standard Appraisals:

Extensive Assessment: Prior to starting TCA treatment, clinicians ought to lead an intensive assessment of the patient's clinical history, including mental history, drug history, substance use, and presence of comorbid ailments.

Actual Assessment: A thorough actual assessment ought to be performed to survey imperative signs, cardiovascular status, neurological capability, and other important boundaries.

Lab Examinations: Benchmark research center tests might incorporate total blood count (CBC), electrolytes, renal capability tests, liver capability tests, and an electrocardiogram (ECG) to survey pattern cardiovascular capability and distinguish any previous irregularities.

Continuous Observing:
Clinical Reaction: Patients ought to be observed consistently for clinical reaction to TCA treatment, including appraisal of

burdensome side effects, utilitarian status, and in general prosperity. Clinicians ought to ask about changes in mind-set, rest, hunger, energy level, and self-destructive ideation.

Antagonistic Impacts: Ordinary checking for unfriendly impacts of TCAs is fundamental to expeditiously identify and oversee likely secondary effects. Patients ought to be taught about normal aftereffects, including anticholinergic impacts, sedation, orthostatic hypotension, and weight gain.

Security Observing: Close checking for indications of suicidality, unsettling, fretfulness, and actuation is essential, particularly during the underlying long stretches of treatment and following portion changes. Patients and parental figures ought to be taught about the advance notice indications of self-destructive ideation and educated to look for sure fire clinical consideration assuming such side effects arise.

Security Insurances:
Self destruction Hazard Evaluation: Clinicians ought to lead an exhaustive self destruction risk evaluation prior to starting TCA treatment, especially in high-risk populaces like youths, youthful grown-ups, and patients with a background marked by self-destructive way of behaving. Close observing for self-destructive ideation and conduct is fundamental all through treatment.

Orthostatic Crucial Signs: Given the gamble of orthostatic hypotension with TCAs, patients ought to be told to screen their pulse and pulse routinely, particularly while changing from deceiving standing positions. Unsteadiness, discombobulation, or syncope ought to be expeditiously answered to medical services suppliers.

Electrocardiographic Checking: Gauge and occasional ECG checking might be shown, particularly in patients with previous cardiovascular circumstances, more seasoned grown-ups, and those getting high TCA portions, to survey for QT prolongation and heart conduction anomalies.

The executives of Unfriendly Occasions:

Suggestive Treatment: The administration of unfavorable occasions related with TCAs might include indicative treatment to lighten explicit side effects. For instance, anticholinergic incidental effects might be made do with anticholinergic adversaries or portion decrease.

Portion Change: At times, portion change or titration of TCAs might be important to limit secondary effects while keeping up with helpful adequacy. Clinicians ought to adjust the requirement for side effect help with the gamble of unfriendly impacts while changing TCA portions.

Drug Connections: Clinicians ought to be careful for potential medication associations that might potentiate or decrease the impacts of TCAs, especially with corresponding utilization of other psychotropic meds, cardiovascular medications, or substances influencing cytochrome P450 catalysts. Portion changes or elective treatments might be justified to moderate the gamble of collaborations.

Patient Instruction and Directing:

Patient schooling is central in TCA treatment to advance medicine adherence, improve patient comprehension of treatment objectives and assumptions, and engage patients to speedily perceive and report antagonistic occasions.

Patients ought to be instructed about the significance of sticking to endorsed dosing regimens, keeping away from unexpected end of TCAs, and looking for clinical consideration in the event that they experience deteriorating side effects or painful aftereffects.

In synopsis, checking and wellbeing contemplations are basic parts of TCA treatment to guarantee ideal treatment results while limiting the gamble of unfavorable impacts and complexities. Clinicians ought to lead careful benchmark evaluations, carry out customary observing conventions, utilize security insurances, and give patient training to alleviate gambles and advance protected and successful TCA treatment. By intently checking patients' clinical reaction, tending to potential antagonistic occasions speedily, and cultivating open correspondence with patients, clinicians can streamline the security and viability of TCA treatment in mental practice.

Chapter Seven

Switching and Discontinuation

Exchanging and end of tricyclic antidepressants (TCAs) require cautious thought to guarantee a smooth change while limiting the gamble of withdrawal side effects and backslide of burdensome side effects. This exhaustive outline will investigate the different parts of changing from TCAs to different antidepressants or ending TCA treatment through and through, including signs for exchanging or cessation, procedures for tightening, the executives of withdrawal side effects, and contemplations for elective medicines.

Signs for Exchanging or Stopping:

Lacking Reaction: Patients who don't accomplish adequate side effect improvement with TCAs might expect changing to elective antidepressants with an alternate component of activity or increase procedures to upgrade viability.

Aftereffects: Excruciating aftereffects or security concerns related with TCAs, like anticholinergic impacts, sedation, orthostatic hypotension, or cardiotoxicity, may require changing to elective meds with a better incidental effect profile.

Drug Connections: Corresponding utilization of TCAs with different drugs that communicate altogether might incite changing to elective antidepressants to keep away from potential pharmacokinetic or pharmacodynamic connections.

Patient Inclination: Patient inclination or adherence issues might impact the choice to switch antidepressants, especially in the event that patients express disappointment with TCA treatment or experience trouble sticking to treatment because of aftereffects or dosing routine.

Methodologies for Exchanging:

Cross-Tapering: Cross-tightening includes continuously tightening the TCA while at the same time starting the new upper to limit cessation side effects and guarantee a smooth change. The pace of cross-tightening relies upon the pharmacokinetic properties of the TCAs and the new energizer.

Tightening Timetable: The tightening timetable ought to be individualized in view of the patient's clinical reaction, decency, and pharmacological properties of the prescriptions in question. A continuous tightening routine more than a little while to months is normally prescribed to diminish the gamble of withdrawal side effects.

Monitoring: Close checking of patients during the exchanging system is fundamental to evaluate for arising withdrawal side effects, screen for helpful reaction to the new stimulant, and change dosing on a case by case basis to upgrade treatment results.

The executives of Withdrawal Side effects:

Withdrawal side effects might happen upon end of TCAs, especially on the off chance that the tightening system is excessively quick or on the other hand if the patient has been on high portions or long haul treatment.

Normal withdrawal side effects might incorporate influenza like side effects (e.g., sickness, migraine, exhaustion), gastrointestinal unsettling influences, dazedness, a sleeping disorder, nervousness, peevishness, and temperament changes.

The board of withdrawal side effects might include indicative treatment with steady measures, like hydration, rest, and non-prescription drugs to lighten explicit side effects.

At times, brief restoration of the TCA or cross-tightening with a more extended acting TCA might be important to oversee serious withdrawal side effects prior to finishing the progress to the new upper.

Contemplations for Elective Medicines:

In the event that changing from TCAs isn't doable or on the other hand assuming patients have encountered different treatment disappointments with different antidepressants, elective treatment choices might be thought of.

Elective medicines might incorporate expansion systems with other psychotropic prescriptions (e.g., abnormal antipsychotics, mind-set stabilizers, lithium), psychotherapy (e.g., mental conduct treatment, relational treatment), electroconvulsive treatment (ECT), or novel medicines like ketamine or transcranial attractive feeling (TMS).

The determination of elective medicines ought to be directed by individual patient qualities, treatment history, comorbidities, and inclinations, fully intent on accomplishing ideal treatment reaction and working on in general utilitarian results.

Patient Instruction and Directing:

Patients going through exchanging or stopping of TCAs ought to get far reaching instruction and directing in regards to the purposes behind the change, the expected course of treatment, and the likely dangers and advantages of elective treatments.

Patients ought to be taught about the chance of withdrawal side effects, the significance of sticking to the recommended tightening routine, and the need to quickly report any disturbing side effects or antagonistic impacts during the change time frame.

Open correspondence among patients and medical care suppliers is vital for address patient worries, ease tension about therapy changes, and encourage cooperation in the therapy dynamic cycle.

In outline, exchanging and cessation of tricyclic antidepressants (TCAs) require cautious preparation, individualized tightening regimens, and close checking to limit the gamble of withdrawal side effects and guarantee a smooth change to elective medicines. Medical care suppliers ought to consider the signs for exchanging or end, utilize proper tightening methodologies, oversee withdrawal side effects proactively, and include patients in shared decision-production to upgrade therapy results and work on quiet fulfillment with energizer treatment.

Chapter Eight

Drug Interactions and Contraindications

Tricyclic antidepressants (TCAs) are related with a critical potential for drug communications because of their complex pharmacokinetic profile and cooperations with different synapse frameworks. Understanding potential medication connections and contraindications is fundamental for clinicians to improve TCA treatment, limit gambles, and guarantee patient security. This exhaustive outline will investigate the components of medication associations with TCAs, normal medication cooperations, contraindications, and procedures for overseeing collaborations in clinical practice.

Instruments of Medication Connections:

Pharmacokinetic Cooperations: TCAs go through broad hepatic digestion by means of the cytochrome P450 (CYP) chemical framework, especially CYP2D6 and CYP2C19 isoenzymes. Drug associations might happen through restraint or acceptance of these chemicals, changing TCA digestion and plasma focuses.

Pharmacodynamic Collaborations: TCAs apply pharmacological impacts through restraint of synapse reuptake, principally serotonin and norepinephrine. Co-organization of different medications that influence synapse frameworks might potentiate or lessen the impacts of TCAs, prompting added substance or adversarial associations.

Normal Medication Communications:

a. Cytochrome P450 Inhibitors:

Specific Serotonin Reuptake Inhibitors (SSRIs): Co-organization of SSRIs with TCAs might expand TCA plasma fixations by hindering CYP2D6-interceded digestion, prompting improved upper impacts and an expanded gamble of secondary effects or poisonousness.

CYP2D6 Inhibitors: Drugs that repress CYP2D6 movement, like fluoxetine, paroxetine, and bupropion, may build TCA plasma focuses and potentiate their belongings.

b. Cytochrome P450 Inducers:

CYP2D6 Inducers: Drugs that prompt CYP2D6 action, for example, carbamazepine, phenytoin, and rifampin, may speed up TCA digestion and lessen plasma fixations, possibly decreasing stimulant viability.

c. Anticholinergic Specialists:

Attendant utilization of TCAs with different meds having anticholinergic properties, like allergy medicines, antipsychotics, antiparkinsonian specialists, and bladder antispasmodics, may build the gamble of anticholinergic secondary effects, including dry mouth, blockage, urinary maintenance, and mental debilitation.

d. Cardiovascular Prescriptions:

QT-Drawing out Specialists: TCAs might draw out the QT span on electrocardiogram (ECG), and accompanying use with other QT-delaying prescriptions, like specific antiarrhythmics, antipsychotics, and antimicrobial specialists (e.g., macrolides, fluoroquinolones), may build the gamble of ventricular arrhythmias.

e. Monoamine Oxidase Inhibitors (MAOIs):

Attending utilization of TCAs with MAOIs is contraindicated because of the gamble of serotonin disorder, hypertensive emergency, and serious unfriendly responses. A waste of time of something like fourteen days is normally suggested between cessation of MAOIs and commencement of TCAs or the other way around.

Contraindications:

a. Extreme touchiness: TCAs are contraindicated in patients with a known touchiness or sensitivity to TCAs or any of their parts.

b. Intense Recuperation Period of Myocardial Localized necrosis: TCAs are contraindicated in patients in the intense recuperation period of myocardial dead tissue because of the gamble of heart arrhythmias and unfriendly cardiovascular impacts.

c. Accompanying Use with MAOIs: As referenced, attendant utilization of TCAs with

MAOIs is contraindicated because of the gamble of serotonin condition, hypertensive emergency, and extreme antagonistic responses.

d. Point Conclusion Glaucoma: TCAs are contraindicated in patients with untreated point conclusion glaucoma because of the potential for worsening of intraocular tension and intense glaucoma assaults.

The board Systems:
Complete Prescription Audit: Clinicians ought to direct an intensive survey of patients'

medicine profiles, including professionally prescribed meds, non-prescription medications, natural enhancements, and dietary enhancements, to distinguish potential medication collaborations with TCAs.

Portion Change: Contingent upon the seriousness of medication associations and the clinical situation, portion changes of TCAs or co-managed drugs might be important to limit gambles and improve treatment results.

Monitoring: Close checking of patients for

unfavorable impacts, helpful reaction, and changes in clinical status is fundamental when TCAs are co-regulated with different prescriptions, especially those known to associate with TCAs.

Think about Elective Treatments: At times, elective treatment choices with a lower hazard of medication cooperations might be thought of, especially in the event that patients have a background marked by critical medication connections or are taking various meds with possible communications.

In rundown, drug associations and contraindications are significant contemplations in the utilization of tricyclic antidepressants (TCAs) to limit gambles and guarantee patient wellbeing. Clinicians ought to know about possible systems of medication cooperations, normal collaborations with TCAs, contraindications to TCA treatment, and procedures for overseeing connections in clinical practice. Far reaching medicine audits, portion changes, observing, and thought of elective treatments are fundamental parts of protected and compelling TCA treatment in mental practice.

Chapter Nine

Patient Education and Counseling in Tricyclic Antidepressant (TCA) Therapy

Patient schooling and directing assume an essential part in improving treatment results, guaranteeing medicine adherence, and advancing patient security in tricyclic energizer (TCA) treatment. Compelling correspondence between medical care suppliers and patients is crucial for upgrade patient comprehension of their condition, therapy choices, likely secondary effects, and self-administration procedures. This extensive outline will investigate the significance of patient schooling and advising in TCA treatment, key parts of patient training, guiding methodologies, and the job of medical care suppliers in cultivating patient commitment and strengthening.

Significance of Patient Instruction:

a. Treatment Getting it: Patient instruction plans to furnish patients with a reasonable comprehension of their condition, including the idea of sadness or other mental issues, the reasoning for TCA treatment, and the normal advantages of treatment.

b. **Medicine Information:** Patients ought to be instructed about the system of activity of TCAs, measurement regimens, possible aftereffects, drug cooperations, and contraindications to guarantee protected and powerful prescription use.

c. **Adherence Advancement:** Patient training assumes a crucial part in advancing drug adherence by tending to misguided judgments, tending to worries, and giving functional procedures to improve adherence, for example, laying out an everyday medicine routine and using adherence helps.

d. Side effect Acknowledgment: Patients ought to be instructed about the signs and side effects of discouragement, possible advance notice indications of demolishing side effects or unfriendly impacts, and when to look for clinical consideration.

e. Self-Administration Abilities: Patient training enables patients to effectively take part in their treatment by showing self-administration abilities, survival techniques, and way of life adjustments to help generally prosperity and side effect the executives.

Key Parts of Patient Schooling:

a. **Individualized Approach:** Patient instruction ought to be custom-made to the singular patient's necessities, inclinations, wellbeing proficiency level, and social foundation to guarantee significance and viability.

b. **Clear Correspondence:** Medical care suppliers ought to utilize clear, language free language and stay away from clinical wording to work with patient comprehension of mind boggling ideas connected with melancholy and TCA treatment.

c. Intelligent Learning: Intelligent instructive strategies, like visual guides, composed materials, interactive media assets, and pretending works out, can upgrade patient commitment and perception of key ideas.

d. Support of Inquiries: Patients ought to be urged to get clarification on some pressing issues, express worries, and effectively partake in treatment decision-production to cultivate a cooperative patient-supplier relationship and advance shared navigation.

e. Support: Patient training ought to be built up at each clinical experience, with amazing open doors for survey, explanation, and support of key messages to improve maintenance and adherence to treatment proposals.

Directing Techniques:
a. Compassion and Backing: Medical services suppliers ought to exhibit sympathy, empathy, and understanding while examining delicate points connected with

emotional well-being and medicine use to establish a steady helpful climate.

b. Psychosocial Evaluation: Directing meetings ought to incorporate a far reaching psychosocial evaluation to recognize factors adding to sadness, survey psychosocial stressors, and investigate patient inclinations and treatment objectives.

c. Psychoeducation: Psychoeducation includes giving patients data about sadness, its causes, side effects, and treatment choices, remembering the job of

TCAs for overseeing burdensome side effects.

d. Mental Conduct Procedures: Mental conduct methods, for example, mental rebuilding, critical thinking abilities preparing, and social enactment, might be integrated into guiding meetings to address maladaptive considerations and ways of behaving related with sorrow.

e. Backslide Anticipation: Patients ought to be instructed about methodologies for forestalling backslide, including adherence to prescription, support of sound way of life propensities, ordinary subsequent arrangements, and early acknowledgment of caution indications of backslide.

Job of Medical services Suppliers:

a. Patient-Focused Care: Medical services suppliers ought to embrace a patient-focused approach that regards patients' independence, inclinations, and therapy objectives, including patients as dynamic members in their consideration.

b. Social Responsiveness: Medical care suppliers ought to show social capability and aversion to address different patient requirements and inclinations, taking into account social convictions, values, and practices that might impact therapy choices.

c. Coherence of Care: Viable correspondence and joint effort between medical services suppliers, including specialists, essential consideration doctors, drug specialists, and emotional well-being experts, are fundamental to guarantee coherence of care and backing all through the therapy cycle.

d. Continuous Help: Medical services suppliers ought to offer continuous help, consolation, and consolation to patients all through their therapy process, addressing any worries or boundaries to adherence that might emerge.

In synopsis, patient training and directing are basic parts of TCA treatment to improve treatment results, advance prescription adherence, and enable patients to partake in their consideration effectively. By giving thorough training, clear correspondence, sympathetic help, and guiding methodologies custom fitted to individual patient requirements, medical care suppliers can work with informed navigation, encourage patient commitment, and work on quiet results in TCA treatment.

Chapter Ten

Future Directions and Research

Tricyclic antidepressants (TCAs) have been a foundation of discouragement treatment for a really long time, exhibiting viability in overseeing burdensome side effects. Nonetheless, progressing research endeavors keep on investigating new roads for further developing TCA treatment, improving treatment results, and tending to existing restrictions. This far reaching outline will investigate latest things, arising research regions, and future bearings in TCA treatment, including pharmacological developments, customized medication draws near, novel treatment systems, and expected regions for future examination.

Pharmacological Advancements:

a. Novel TCA Subsidiaries: Research endeavors are in progress to foster novel TCA subsidiaries with improved pharmacokinetic profiles, upgraded receptor selectivity, and decreased aftereffects contrasted with conventional TCAs. These mixtures might offer better bearableness and viability in overseeing burdensome side effects.

b. Designated Medication Conveyance Frameworks: Propels in drug conveyance innovation, like nanotechnology and designated drug conveyance frameworks, may work with the advancement of TCA details with further developed bioavailability, tissue explicitness, and supported discharge properties, enhancing remedial adequacy and limiting unfavorable impacts.

Customized Medication Approaches:

a. Pharmacogenomics: Pharmacogenomic concentrates on expect to recognize hereditary biomarkers related with individual changeability in TCA reaction and vulnerability to unfavorable impacts. Fitting TCA treatment in light of patients' hereditary profiles might empower customized treatment draws near, upgrading restorative results and limiting dangers.

b. Biomarkers: Research endeavors center around distinguishing fringe and neuroimaging biomarkers related with treatment reaction, reduction, and backslide in TCA treatment. Biomarker-directed treatment procedures might work with early distinguishing proof of treatment non-responders and illuminate customized treatment choices.

Novel Treatment Techniques:

a. Mix Treatments: Investigational studies investigate the viability and wellbeing of blend treatments including TCAs and other pharmacological specialists, like abnormal antipsychotics, temperament stabilizers, or glutamatergic modulators. Blend treatments might focus on different synapse frameworks and proposition synergistic impacts in overseeing treatment-safe wretchedness.

b. Increase Systems: Research centers around recognizing novel expansion techniques to upgrade TCA adequacy in treatment-safe sadness, including non-pharmacological mediations like ketamine imbuement treatment, transcranial attractive excitement (TMS), or psychotherapy modalities.

Advanced Wellbeing Intercessions:

a. Portable Wellbeing (mHealth) Applications: Arising research investigates the practicality and adequacy of mHealth mediations, for example, cell phone applications and wearable gadgets, in supporting TCA adherence, observing burdensome side effects, and working with distant patient-supplier correspondence.

b. Telepsychiatry: Telepsychiatry administrations offer remote admittance to psychological well-being care, empowering patients to get TCA treatment, psychoeducation, and directing administrations by means of telecom advances. Telepsychiatry might further develop admittance to mind, especially in underserved or distant regions, and upgrade treatment adherence and commitment.

Neurobiological Components:
   a. Neuroinflammation: Preclinical and clinical examinations research the job of neuroinflammation and resistant dysregulation in sadness pathophysiology and TCA reaction. Focusing on neuroinflammatory pathways

might address a clever helpful way to deal with upgrade TCA viability and further develop treatment results.

b. Brain adaptability: Research endeavors center around clarifying the brain adaptability instruments basic TCA-interceded energizer impacts, including synaptic renovating, neurogenesis, and synapse receptor regulation. Upgrading brain adaptability might offer novel restorative focuses for creating cutting edge antidepressants.

Relative Adequacy Exploration:

a. Similar Adequacy and Bearableness: Near adequacy concentrates on plan to assess the relative viability, wellbeing, and bearableness of TCAs contrasted with other upper classes, including specific serotonin reuptake inhibitors (SSRIs), serotonin-norepinephrine reuptake inhibitors (SNRIs), and more current age antidepressants.

b. Long haul Results: Longitudinal examinations research the drawn out viability, strength of reaction, and backslide counteraction methodologies in

TCA-treated patients, giving significant bits of knowledge into the ideal term of TCA treatment and techniques for keeping up with abatement.

In rundown, future headings and examination in TCA treatment envelop a different scope of regions, including pharmacological developments, customized medication draws near, novel treatment methodologies, computerized wellbeing mediations, neurobiological systems, and relative viability research. By utilizing arising innovations, propelling comprehension we might interpret sadness pathophysiology, and taking on a customized way to deal with treatment, future examination attempts hold the possibility to upgrade TCA treatment's viability, decency, and openness, eventually further developing results for patients with gloom and related mental issues.

www.ingramcontent.com/pod-product-compliance
Lightning Source LLC
Chambersburg PA
CBHW070145230526
45471CB00002B/523